CISSN & IS Study Guide

Jose Antonio PhD
FISSN FNSCA CSCS

issn
international society of sports nutrition

Dedication

To my daughters who grew up to be smarter than I

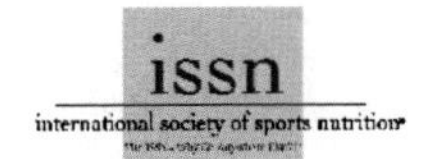

TABLE OF CONTENTS

issn

international society of sports nutrition

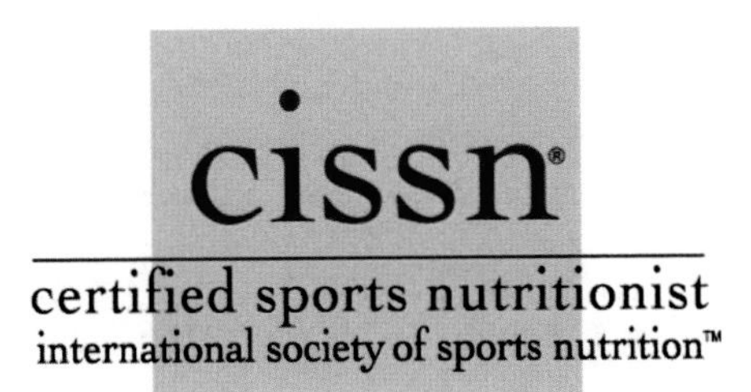

The CISSN is our advanced sports nutrition certification.

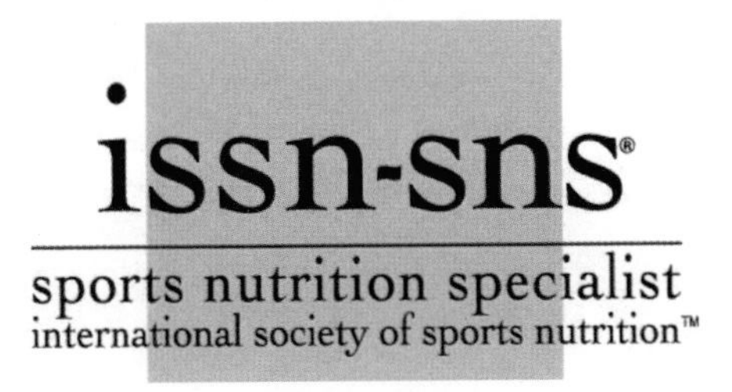

The ISSN-SNS is our introductory sports nutrition certification. Please visit www.issn.net for more details on the ISSN and our certifications.

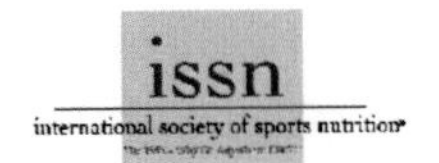

Quick Note (because nobody ever reads the Preface):

There are several books that can be used as a reference for the CISSN and ISSN-SNS Exams. These include:

- **Sports Nutrition & Performance Enhancing Supplements. Eds. Abbie Smith-Ryan PhD and Jose Antonio PhD. ISBN: 1-60797-339-1. Linus Books. 2013. (Note:** *this study guide is largely modeled after this book; however, you can get the information needed to answer the questions in the Study Guide from the resources listed below***).**
- Essentials of Sports Nutrition and Supplements. Antonio, J.; Kalman, D.; Stout, J.R.; Greenwood, M.; Willoughby, D.S.; Haff, G.G. (Eds.) 2008, Approx. 875 p. 123 illus. With CD-ROM., Hardcover, ISBN: 978-1-58829-611-5.
- Dietary Protein and Resistance Exercise. Eds. Lonnie Michael Lowery and Jose Antonio. 2012. CRC Press.
- Exercise & Sport Nutrition: Principles, Promises, Science & Recommendations. Authors: Richard Kreider, Brian Leutholtz, Frank Katch and Victor Katch. Publisher: Fitness Technologies Press. ISBN-10: 0974296562 2009.
- Nutritional Supplements in Sports and Exercise 2nd edition by Mike Greenwood, Matthew Cooke, Tim Ziegenfuss, Douglas Kalman and Jose Antonio. (2015).

The CISSN and ISSN-SNS Study Guide uses information from these books, the ISSN Position Papers (http://www.biomedcentral.com/collections/ISSNPosP), and pertinent peer-reviewed science found in various journals. Either way, if you use this study guide thoroughly, you should pass the certifications (either one).

Important: You will see that much of the Study Guide will have references throughout. Those references are there to assist you in answering the questions posed.

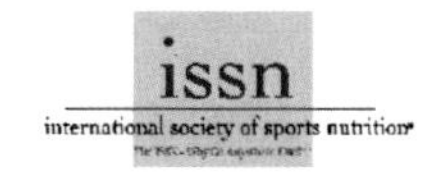

Chapter 1 – BIOENERGETICS and SKELETAL MUSCLE[1-4,5]

EXERCISE 1

1. The structure of ATP is one that contains:
   a. A nitrogenous purine base, hexose sugar and three phosphates.
   b. A nitrogenous purine base, glucose and two phosphates.
   c. A carbohydrate base, pentose sugar and three phosphates.
   d. A nitrogenous purine base, pentose sugar and three phosphates.
2. The process of skeletal muscle differentiation is controlled by four highly related basic helix-loop helix proteins referred to as the myogenic regulatory factors or MRFs. These include:
   a. Myo-D, myogenin, MRF-4, and myf5.
   b. Myo-D, myogenin, MRF-4, and myostatin.
   c. Myosin heavy chain, myogenin, MRF-4, and myf5.
   d. Myo-D, myogenin, titin, and myf5.
3. The three primary energy systems used by the human body includes:
   a. Phosphagen, Aerobic, and Lactic Acid
   b. Pyruvic Acid, Aerobic, and Lactic Acid
   c. Phosphagen, Aerobic, and Beta-Oxidation
   d. Phosphagen, Transaminase, and Lactic Acid
4. The three skeletal muscle fiber types found in humans include:
   a. Type I, IIA and IIX
   b. Type IIA, IIX and III
   c. Type I, II, III
   d. Type I, IID, IIX
5. The primary energy system used during the 60 meter dash is:
   a. ATP-PCr
   b. Lactic Acid
   c. Aerobic
   d. All are used equally
6. Which of the following energy systems are predominant in the 10,000 meter track race?
   a. ATP-PCr

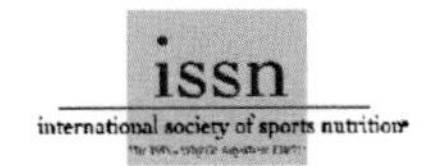

   b. Lactic Acid
   c. Aerobic
   d. All are used equally

7. Short-duration, high-intensity exercise (i.e., longer than 20 seconds) relies on __________ as well as stored ______ to a lesser extent.
   a. Fast glycolysis, triglycerides
   b. Beta-oxidation, phosphagens
   c. Fast glycolysis, phosphagens
   d. Slow glycolysis, phosphagens
8. As exercise intensity increases (e.g., running at 50% HRmax to 90% of HRmax)
   a. The % of fat that is oxidized increases
   b. The % of glycogen that is oxidized increases
   c. The role of the ATP-PCr energy system increases
   d. The importance of protein as a fuel source increases
9. The increase in skeletal muscle fiber number seen with various models of overload may be due to:
   a. Muscle fiber splitting and satellite cell inactivation
   b. Satellite cell activation/proliferation and Myostatin promotion.
   c. Satellite cell activation and muscle fiber splitting
   d. There is no evidence that skeletal muscles can increase fiber number
10. Which of the following skeletal muscle fiber types would exhibit the greatest force production?
   a. Type I
   b. Type IIA
   c. Type IIX
   d. Type C

EXERCISE 2

1. Describe three characteristics that are different between Type I, IIA and IIX muscle fibers.

2. Name 3 sports in track and field in which the ATP-PCr (aka Phosphagen energy system) energy system is predominant.

3. Name any 3 sports in which the Lactic Acid (fast glycolysis) energy system predominates.

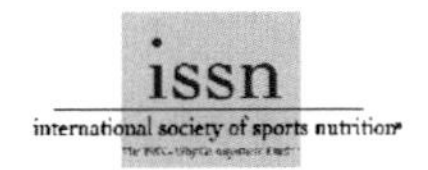

4. Name any 3 sports in which the Aerobic energy system predominates.

5. Describe the role of satellite cells in skeletal muscle.

EXERCISE 3

Match the characteristic with the specific skeletal muscle fiber type. Answer choices include:
A) Slow Twitch or Type I B) Fast Twitch or Type II

1. Greatest muscle fiber diameter ____
2. Lowest mitochondrial density ____
3. Highest concentration of creatine phosphate ____
4. Highest concentration of triglyceride stores ____
5. Highest oxidative enzyme activity ____
6. Fastest contraction speed ____
7. Lowest recruitment threshold ____
8. Largest neuron size ____
9. Highest myoglobin content ____
10. Lowest capillary density ____

Exercise 4

True (A) or False (B)

1. The skeletal muscle fiber type that will be most likely found in the breast muscles of domestic chickens are fast-twitch or Type II.

2. The primary energy system used during a Sumo wrestling match is the aerobic system.

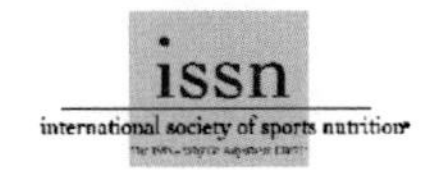

3. When activated, satellite cells can undergo mitosis and may eventually create new or nascent skeletal muscle fibers (i.e., skeletal muscle fiber hyperplasia).

4. The rate-limiting step in glycolysis is at the enzyme, PFK or phosphofructokinase.

5. The primary energy system used during a 400 meter dash is the lactic acid system.

6. Myostatin is a myokine that acts as a negative regulator of skeletal muscle mass.

7. There is a linear relationship between oxygen uptake and heart rate.

8. The primary limiting factor in maximal oxygen uptake (for the vast majority of aerobic exercise) is cardiac output.

9. There is an inverse relationship between volume or duration of exercise and intensity.

10. The primary fuel used during low-level aerobic activity is fat (i.e., free fatty acids).

FUN FACT! *Darryn Willoughby PhD FISSN (Baylor University) does some of the coolest work on the effects of supplements on skeletal muscle using molecular biology techniques. He showed for instance that creatine supplementation upregulates the expression of MHC mRNA.*

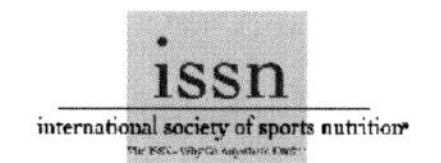

CHAPTER 2 – PROTEIN AND AMINO ACIDS [6-22]

Exercise 1

1. Which of the following dietary components are likely the most important in athletes training for skeletal muscle hypertrophy?
    a. Post workout consumption of protein
    b. Total protein intake (grams per day)
    c. Type of protein consumed
    d. Nighttime feeding of protein
2. Which of the following have been shown to occur in individuals consuming a high protein diet for a 1-year period?
    a. Elevated liver enzymes
    b. Evidence of renal dysfunction
    c. Chronic dehydration
    d. None of the above
3. Which of the following dietary proteins will likely elevate muscle protein synthesis the most when consumed immediately post-workout?
    a. Wheat
    b. Whey
    c. Soy
    d. Rice
4. Which of the following dietary proteins contain the highest concentration of leucine?
    a. Casein
    b. Rice
    c. Whey
    d. Beef
5. Which of the following are known harmful side effects of high protein diets (> 3 grams per kg per day)?
    a. Dehydration
    b. Problems with glomerular filtration
    c. Adrenal fatigue
    d. None of the above
6. Which of the following are functional roles of protein?
    a. Hormones
    b. Enzymes
    c. Growth and Maintenance
    d. All of the above
7. ______________ constitute approximately 33% of skeletal

muscle protein.

a. Valine, leucine and glycine
b. Valine, glycine and asparagine
c. The Branched-Chain Amino Acids
d. Taurine, histidine and glycine

8. The consumption of a high protein diet (~3 g per kg per day) for two months may result in:
   a. A gain in LBM
   b. A loss of fat mass
   c. An elevation of plasma creatinine
   d. Both a and b are correct
9. Amino acids are the building blocks of protein. Which of the following amino acids are considered essential?
   a. Taurine
   b. Glutamine
   c. Cysteine
   d. Lysine
10. The combination of ___________ and supplemental ______ may be useful in the treatment of sarcopenia.
    a. Aerobic exercise, carbohydrate
    b. Resistance exercise, protein
    c. Resistance exercise, sports drinks
    d. Aerobic exercise, protein

Exercise 2

1. According to the work of Macnaughton et al., describe the response of muscle protein synthesis following a 40 versus 20 gram bolus of ingested whey protein.[23]

2. According to the work of Antonio et al., what changes are seen with a high protein diet combined with a periodized resistance training program.[10]

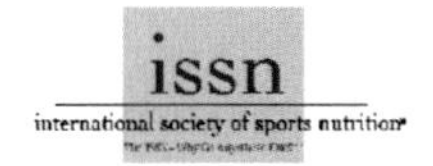

3. Describe briefly the difference between the 'protein spread' versus 'protein change' theory according to Bosse and Dixon.[16]

4. According to Moore et al [24], what are the differences in myofibrillar protein synthesis in older versus younger individuals after consuming protein.

5. The amino acid that is the most important in determining protein quality is ____________.

6. List the essential amino acids.

Exercise 3

True (A) or False (B)

1. The Recommended Dietary Allowance (RDA) for protein intake in adults is 0.8 g/kg/d (https://ods.od.nih.gov/Health_Information/Dietary_Reference_Intakes.aspx/)

2. High protein intakes for a period of one-year (> 2 g/kg/d) have been shown to have no harmful effects on renal function.

3. The thermic effect of protein exceeds that of carbohydrate or fat.

4. Milk protein typically has a higher leucine concentration than non-animal based proteins such as wheat.

5. There is evidence to suggest that in active (aerobic or resistance-trained) individuals, consuming a higher protein diet (> 2 g/kg/d) may result in a decrement of bone mineral content.

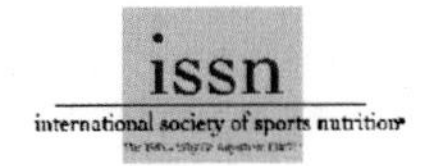

6. In general, head to head comparisons of whey versus soy protein demonstrate that whey is a more potent stimulator of skeletal muscle protein synthesis.

7. Older individuals have lower rates of protein synthesis in response to protein feeding and thus will likely require more protein than a younger individual.

8. Daily overfeeding on carbohydrate + fat versus protein alone has similar effects in terms of body fat gains (assuming feedings are isocaloric).

9. Glutamine is considered a conditionally essential amino acid.

10. The branched-chain amino acids are comprised of leucine, valine and isoleucine.

FUN FACT! *An RCT from our lab at Nova Southeastern University showed that a 1-year high protein diet had no deleterious effects on hepatic and renal function. Nor did blood lipids change. Yep. Whey protein for everyone!*

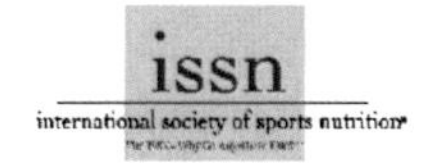

CHAPTER 3 - CARBOHYDRATE

Exercise 1

1. Monosaccharides are the smallest carbohydrate molecules and include ___________.
   a. Glucose
   b. Fructose
   c. Galactose
   d. All of the above are monosaccharides
2. Sucrose is _________ linked to _________and is derived from the sugar cane plant and is often referred to as "table sugar."
   a. Glucose, fructose
   b. Galactose, fructose
   c. Glucose, ribose
   d. Ribose, fructose
3. _____________________ are composed of 3-10 monosaccharides and include stachyose, raffinose, and verbascose.
   a. Monosaccharides
   b. Potatoes
   c. Disaccharides
   d. Oligosaccharides
4. _____________ is the building block of plant starch. Straight chains of starch are referred to as _________, and branched chains of amylose are referred to as amylopectin.
   a. Glucose, amylose
   b. Sucrose, amylose
   c. Deoxyribose, pectin
   d. Glucose, fiber
5. Glycogen, made up of branched chains of glucose, is produced and stored primarily in the _________and _____________.
   a. Liver, skeletal muscle
   b. Liver, kidneys
   c. Cardiac muscle, brain
   d. Kidneys, skeletal muscle
6. There is a _________ relationship between exercise __________ and the rate of skeletal muscle glycogen breakdown.
   a. Weak, intensity
   b. Strong, intensity

c. Strong, mode
d. Weak, mode

7. During the first 30 minutes of moderate to heavy aerobic exercise, most of the glucose output from the liver is derived from ____________________ and not gluconeogenesis.
   a. Food the you have recently consumed
   b. Hepatic glycogen stores
   c. Glycogenesis
   d. Conversion of lactate to glucose
8. Higher levels of pre-exercise glycogen results in a __________ rate of breakdown during exercise.
   a. Marginally slower
   b. Significantly slower
   c. Greater
   d. No effect
9. Moderate submaximal intensity training (such as 60% VO_{2max}) leads to an increase in the glycogen content in skeletal muscle, primarily in ___________ skeletal muscle fibers.
   a. Type I
   b. Type IIA
   c. Type IIX
   d. Type I, IIA and IIX equally
10. Glycogen loading is also known as
    a. Carbohydrate loading
    b. Carb loading
    c. Muscle glycogen supercompensation
    d. All of the above

Exercise 2

1. Describe the 'classic' method of carbohydrate loading.

2. Describe the acute effects of carbohydrate supplementation on intermittent sports performance.[25]

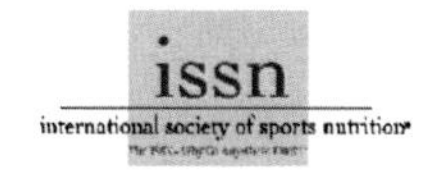

3. Give a brief summary of the effects of oral carbohydrate rinsing and its effects on performance.[26]

4. Summarize briefly the amount of carbohydrate needed to enhance endurance exercise capacity.[27]

5. Describe some of the myths and misconceptions surrounding carbohydrate feeding pre-exercise.[28]

Exercise 3

Approximately how many grams of carbohydrate are needed for the duration of exercise listed below?[29]

1. 2-3 hours of exercise
2. ultraendurance events

Exercise 4
True (A) or False (B)

1. Sucrose is a simple sugar formed from glucose and fructose.

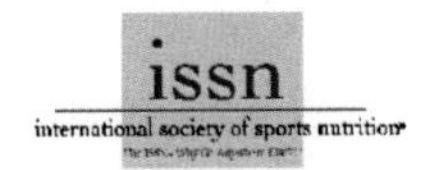

2. Complex carbohydrates include both fiber and starches. These include foods such as potatoes, grains, and other plant foods.

3. The timing, dosage and type of carbohydrate consumed during a prolonged endurance event can have a significant effect on performance.

4. The elevation in plasma insulin after the consumption of carbohydrate-containing foods is the primary reason individuals gain body weight and fat.

5. As exercise intensity increases, the primary fuel used is carbohydrate (over free fatty acids).

FUN FACT! *Work by Asker Jeukendrup PhD has shown that you can oxidize as much as 105 grams of carbohydrate per hour during exercise! Now that's a lot of sugar. Cinnabons for everyone!*

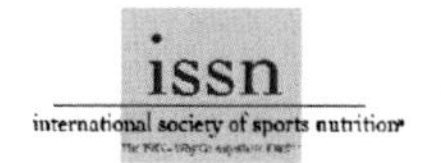

CHAPTER 4 - FAT

Exercise 1

1. The triglyceride or triacylglycerol molecule is composed of
    a. A ribose backbone and three fatty acids
    b. A fatty acid backbone and three glycerol molecules
    c. A glycerol backbone and three fatty acids
    d. A glycerol backbone and conjugated linoleic acid
2. The primary fuel at rest is
    a. Triglycerides
    b. Cholesterol
    c. Phospholipids
    d. Glycerol
3. The RER or respiratory exchange ratio of an individual that is mainly oxidizing fat would be
    a. Close to 0.9
    b. Greater than 1.0
    c. Close to 0.7
    d. Exactly 0.85
4. Eicosapentaenoic acid (EPA) and docosahexanoic acid (DHA) are examples of which type of fatty acid?
    a. Omega-3
    b. Omega-6
    c. Omega-9
    d. Omega-13
5. Trained aerobic athletes have a greater ability to oxidize fat due to
    a. Increased mitochondrial volume and density
    b. Increased percentage of type IIX skeletal muscle fibers
    c. Decreased myoglobin
    d. All of the above
6. Fatty acids
    a. Are basically hydrocarbon chains of varying lengths
    b. Can be saturated or unsaturated
    c. Are an essential part of one's diet
    d. All of the above
7. What are the essential fatty acids that humans need in their diet since they do not make them endogenously?
    a. EPA and linoleic acid
    b. EPA and DHA
    c. CLA and ALA

d. Linoleic acid and linolenic acid

8. In the resting *fed state* (e.g. after consuming a mixed meal), RER will
    a. Typically rise
    b. Typically decrease
    c. Remain neutral
    d. Typically drop to 0.6
9. Which of the following exercises will preferentially oxidize fat as fuel during the event itself?
    a. 10 k run
    b. 100 meter dash
    c. Hiking at an easy pace for 3 hours
    d. Doing 10 sets of 10 reps of the back squat
10. Regarding maximal fat oxidation (MFO), which of the following are true?[30]
    a. MFO is higher in women than men (when expressed per unit FFM)
    b. MFO is higher in soccer players than American football players
    c. Male athletes are higher than female athletes (when expressed in absolute terms)
    d. All of the above

Exercise 2

1. According to the work of Randell et al., describe the range of maximal fat oxidation in athletes, any sex differences, as well as differences between sports.[30]

2. Explain briefly the differences in fat oxidation between rowing and cycling across a range of exercise intensities.[31]

3. Explain briefly the effects of omega 3 fatty acid supplementation for 12 weeks on a group of healthy older females.[32]

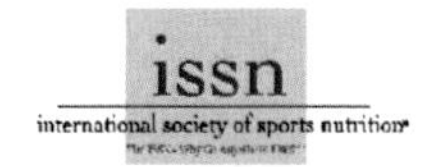

4. Overall, what does the scientific literature indicate regarding the effects of CLA supplementation on measures of body composition?[33, 34]

5. Describe the body composition alterations that occur in a fed vs. fasted state after aerobic exercise training.[35]

Exercise 3

True (A) or False (B)

1. Fat has a many roles in the human body. They include serving as part of the cell membrane, the formation of hormones and as a storage form of energy.

2. The term "omega-3" (in reference to fish fat, specifically omega-3 fatty acids) refers to the fact that there is a C=C double bond at the third carbon from the end of the hydrocarbon chain.

3. The two essential fatty acids are linoleic and alpha-linolenic acid.

4. At the same absolute workload, endurance-trained individuals will preferentially oxidize more fat than an untrained individual.

5. There is a significant body of evidence which clearly demonstrates that consuming saturated fat can increase the risk of cardiovascular disease.

6. The primary fuel during the resting state is free fatty acids.

7. Training in a fasted state has been shown to promote a greater level of fatty acid oxidation.

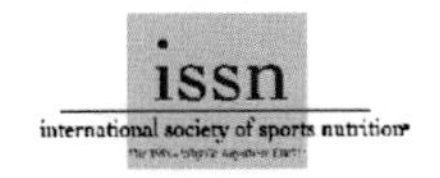

8. Omega-3 fatty acids have been shown to have anti-inflammatory properties.

9. Avocadoes and almonds are excellent sources of monounsaturated fat.

10. Saturated fat molecules contain no C=C double bonds (carbon to carbon).

FUN FACT! *Did you know that maximal fat oxidation is greater in women compared to men (expressed relative to FFM), according to Randell et al. Now that's cool. Ok ladies. Go oxidize some fat.*

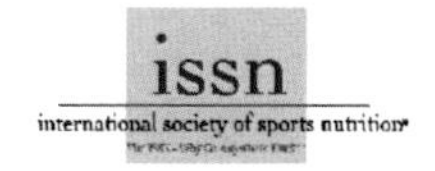

CHAPTER 5 - CREATINE[36-40]

Exercise 1

1. Creatine supplementation plus resistance exercise increases _________ and strength. Based on the magnitude inferences it appears that consuming creatine immediately post-workout is ________ to pre-workout vis a vis body composition and strength.[37]
    a. Fat mass, inferior
    b. Fat-free mass, superior
    c. Organ mass, superior
    d. Fat-free mass, inferior
2. Short-term data has shown that supplementation of creatine nitrate[41]
    a. Is well-tolerated and can significantly increase skeletal muscle creatine concentration
    b. Is not well tolerated but can significantly increase skeletal muscle creatine concentration
    c. Is ineffectual in elevating skeletal muscle creatine concentration
    d. None of the above are true
3. Creatine was first discovered through meat extraction in the 1830s by French scientist
    a. Jacques Cousteau
    b. Michel Eugene Chevreul
    c. Louis Pasteur
    d. Rene Descartes
4. The ____________, ______________, and ________ are the primary sites of its endogenous creatine synthesis, utilizing the amino acids arginine, glycine, and methionine as precursors in its production.
    a. Liver, kidney, pituitary gland
    b. Liver, adipose tissue, pancreas
    c. Liver, kidney, brain
    d. Liver, kidney, pancreas
5. The overwhelming majority (~95%) of Cr is stored within _______________ cells, while the remaining amounts (~5%) are found within the brain, eye, kidneys and _____.[42, 43].
    a. Skeletal muscle, spleen
    b. Spleen, skeletal muscle
    c. Skeletal muscle, testes
    d. Skeletal muscle, penis

6. In un-supplemented individuals, the body's pool of creatine is approximately ____ grams. It is maintained through a combination of dietary intake and organ synthesis.
    a. 0.1
    b. 2
    c. 5
    d. 10
7. Which of the following foods would likely have the highest concentration of creatine?
    a. Milk
    b. Herring
    c. Beef
    d. Wheat
8. Which of these are possible ergogenic effects of creatine supplementation?
    a. Increased LBM
    b. Increased strength
    c. Increased muscular endurance
    d. All of the above
9. The combination of Cr and ____________ has been shown to promote elevations in skeletal muscle glycogen concentrations, better than carbohydrate loading alone.[44, 45]
    a. Fatty acids
    b. Lipoic acid
    c. Carbohydrate
    d. None of the above
10. The typical 'maintenance' dose of creatine is
    a. 1-2 grams
    b. 3-5 grams
    c. 10-15 grams
    d. 15-20 grams

Exercise 2

1. Describe the typical loading protocol for creatine.

2. Creatine is made from which three amino acids?

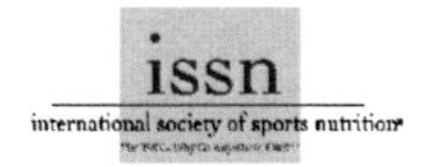

3. How does creatine supplementation affect meat-eaters vs. vegetarians vis a vis brain function?[46]

4. Describe briefly the effect of creatine supplementation on post-exercise skeletal muscle glycogen storage.[47]

5. List 7 sports from Track and Field events in which creatine supplementation would likely be of benefit.

6. Describe briefly the effects of creatine monohydrate versus creatine ethyl ester.[48]

7. Describe briefly the effects of creatine monohydrate on myosin heavy chain expression.[49]

8. Is there a benefit for creatine supplementation vis a vis muscle disorders?[50]

9. Is there a timing effect (pre versus post exercise) regarding creatine supplementation in healthy older adults?[51]

Exercise 3

True (A) or False (B)

1. Regular supplementation with creatine monohydrate has been shown to deleteriously affect fluid retention.

2. Creatine ethyl ester has been shown to be more effective (for LBM gains) than creatine monohydrate when given at the same absolute dosage.

3. Creatine supplementation has been shown to impact mRNA of type I, IIA and IIX myosin heavy chain isoforms.

4. One of the more common 'side effects' of creatine supplementation is dehydration.

5. Creatine supplementation has been shown to have no harmful effects on renal function.

6. Roughly 95% of the body's creatine stores can be found in skeletal muscles.

7. Creatine is also stored in the brain, liver and kidneys.

8. There is evidence to suggest that supplementing with creatine can improve memory.

9. Vegans will likely respond to creatine supplementation more so than meat-eaters.

10. The food(s) with the highest concentration of creatine is fish.

FUN FACT! *Roger Harris PhD FISSN was one of the very first scientists to test the effects of creatine on skeletal muscle. As of now there are literally hundreds of studies on creatine. Yet it is still the most widely misunderstood supplement. If some self-appointed expert tells you that creatine supplementation causes harm, run the other way. Make sure you recruit your type IIA and IIX skeletal muscle fibers to ensure a quick getaway.*

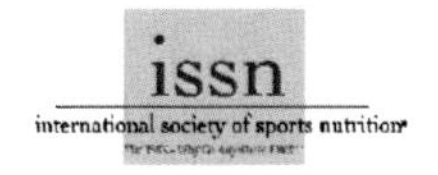

CHAPTER 6 – CAFFEINE[52]

Exercise 1

1. Caffeine is effective for enhancing sport performance in trained athletes when consumed in low-to-moderate dosages (~_______________) and overall does not result in further enhancement in performance when consumed in higher dosages (>/= 9 mg/kg).
    a. 3-6 g of caffeine per kg body weight
    b. 1-2 mg of caffeine per kg body weight
    c. 3-6 mg of caffeine per kg body weight
    d. 1-2 g of caffeine per kg body weight
2. Elevated levels of caffeine can appear in the bloodstream within ___________ minutes of consumption, and peak concentrations are evident _________ post ingestion.
    a. 1-2, 20 minutes
    b. 10-15, 45-60 minutes
    c. 30-45, 100 minutes
    d. 90-120, 3 hours
3. Research suggests that during exercise, caffeine may decrease the reliance on glycogen utilization and increase the ability to utilize _____________ for energy.
    a. Amino acids
    b. Free fatty acids
    c. Ketones
    d. All of the above
4. Which of the following may occur from caffeine intake?
    a. Increased CNS alertness
    b. Enhanced lipolysis
    c. Improved exercise performance
    d. All of the above
5. Caffeine supplementation has been shown to
    a. Lower one's rating of perceived muscle soreness
    b. Improve endurance performance
    c. Improve strength
    d. All of the above
6. Caffeine exerts its effects via
    a. An effect on the CNS
    b. An effect on substrate utilization
    c. An increase in the secretion of beta-endorphins
    d. All of the above
7. Caffeine has been shown to enhance several different modes of exercise performance including:

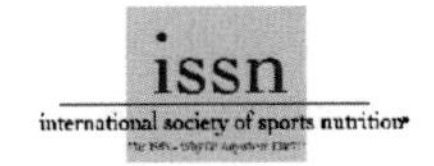

a. Endurance
b. High-intensity team sport activity
c. Strength-power performance
d. All of the above

8. During exercise, the consumption of caffeine may induce
    a. Diuresis
    b. A negative effect on fluid balance
    c. An increase in sweat rate
    d. None of the above
9. Research pertaining exclusively to women is limited; however, studies have shown a ________ for conditioned strength-power female athletes and a moderate _________ in performance for recreationally active women.
    a. Detriment, increase
    b. Benefit, increase
    c. Neutral effect, increase
    d. Benefit, decrease
10. During periods of sleep deprivation, caffeine can act to ______________________, which has been shown to be an effective aid for special operations military personnel, as well as athletes during times of exhaustive exercise that requires sustained focus.
    a. Enhance alertness
    b. Decrease vigilance
    c. Decrease operational effectiveness
    d. None of the above are correct

Exercise 2

1. What is the genotype that will likely benefit the most from caffeine supplementation?[53]

2. Describe the dose response of an energy drink containing caffeine on muscle performance.[54]

3. Describe the effects of combining caffeine with p-synephrine on resistance exercise performance.[55]

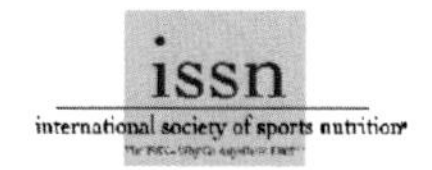

4. List 5 sports in which caffeine may exert an ergogenic effect.

5. Describe briefly the difference in caffeine-habituated vs. caffeine-naïve individuals in terms of the ergogenic effect of the drug.

6. List some of the possible mechanisms by which caffeine exerts an ergogenic effect.

7. What is the recommended dosage of caffeine (range) needed to exert an ergogenic effect.

8. What are some possible side effects from consuming excessive caffeine?

9. Discuss briefly the differences (if any) between coffee and caffeine in terms of their ergogenic effects.[56, 57]

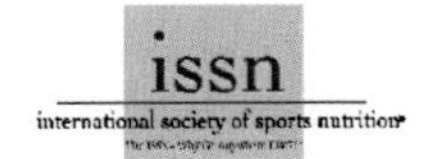

Exercise 3

True (A) or False (B)

1. The single biggest source of anti-oxidants for most individuals is coffee.

2. Symptoms of consuming excessive caffeine include anxiety, insomnia and restlessness.

3. Caffeine functions by blocking the effects of adenosine, leading to less tiredness or fatigue.

4. There is evidence to suggest that caffeine can lower the risk of depression.

5. An effective dose of caffeine for an ergogenic effect is 5 mg per kg body weight.

6. Acute caffeine consumption can elevate metabolic rate as well as enhance fat oxidation.

7. Caffeine is a dehydrating agent.

8. Caffeine is an effective ergogenic aid for endurance sports.

9. One way in which caffeine can enhance exercise performance is by increasing one's pain threshold.

10. Acute caffeine consumption has been shown to improve strength (1-RM).

FUN FACT! *Back in the late 1970s, David Costill PhD did the seminal study showing that caffeine was indeed a super-duper ergogenic aid! Can you actually drink too much coffee? Hmmm...Nah. ☺*

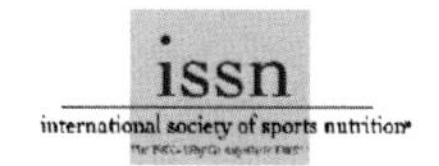

Chapter 7 – Nutrient Timing[58]

Exercise 1

1. Regarding carbohydrate feeding, which of the following strategies would likely have the greatest performance benefit for a 10 km running race?
    a. A high carbohydrate meal the night before
    b. Consuming a high glycemic index carbohydrate immediately pre- and during the race.
    c. Consuming a high carbohydrate meal post-race
    d. All of the above are equally effective
2. Glycogen stores are quite limited in skeletal muscle. Endogenous stores of glycogen may last approximately _________ during moderate to high intensity aerobic exercise.
    a. 1.5 to 3 hours
    b. 10-60 minutes
    c. 3-6 hours
    d. 10-15 hours
3. The preponderance of evidence suggests that the ingestion of _________ during endurance type exercise is a well-established strategy to sustain blood _______ levels, possibly spare glycogen and thus promote greater levels of performance.
    a. Carbohydrate, glucose
    b. Fat, glucose
    c. Ketones, glucose
    d. Carbohydrate, fatty acid
4. Effective nutrient timing strategies involve the possible use of
    a. Protein
    b. Carbohydrate
    c. Caffeine
    d. All of the above
5. A single bout of resistance exercise results in the acute stimulation of MPS or muscle protein synthesis above baseline values. MPS may remain elevated for approximately as long as _________ post exercise.
    a. 3-10 hours
    b. 30 minutes to 3 hours
    c. 48-96 hours
    d. 24-48 hours
6. Another benefit of nutrient timing seen in US Marine

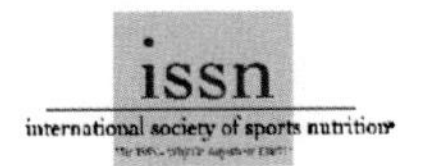

recruits in the immediate post-workout phase includes:[59]
   a. Fewer muscle/joint problems
   b. Less heat exhaustion
   c. Fewer medical visits
   d. All of the above
7. Caffeine can be used to elicit an ergogenic response. An effective timing strategy would be to consume _________ about _________ prior to an intense bout of exercise.
   a. 5 mg/kg, one day
   b. 1 mg/kg, 20-40 minutes
   c. 5 mg/kg, 30-60 minutes
   d. 5 g/kg, 60-120 minutes
8. Which of the following would likely provide the best strategy to promote recovery (i.e., glycogen repletion and enhancement of MPS) after doing 2 hours of aerobic exercise at 70% of HRmax?
   a. 16 ounces of chocolate milk immediately post-exercise
   b. 16 ounces of a traditional sports drink immediately post-exercise
   c. 16 ounces of water immediately post-exercise
   d. Consuming nothing post-exercise is best
9. Which of the following provide a potent MPS response when consumed immediately post-resistance training?
   a. Milk, EAAs and Whey
   b. Milk, Wheat, and Soy
   c. EAAs, Whey and Hemp
   d. None of the above
10. Which of these is clearly an ineffectual nutrient timing strategy to enhance exercise performance?
   a. Consuming 30-60 grams of carbohydrate during the 2nd hour of 3-hour long running race.
   b. Consuming 5 mg/kg of caffeine 30 minutes prior to a half-marathon race.
   c. Consuming 16 ounces water immediately post-exercise (ex. Running in 30 degree C temperatures for 100 minutes).
   d. Consuming 30 grams of a high glycemic index carbohydrate ten minutes prior to a 10k running race.

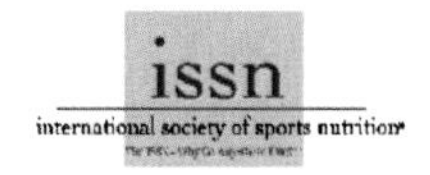

Exercise 2

1. Provide a brief list of sports or activities in which consuming carbohydrate + protein during the peri-workout window may indeed confer a benefit.

2. Describe which nutrient timing strategy was superior (Pulse, Intermediate or Bolus) in the paper by Areta et al.[60]

3. In the paper by Kanda et al., describe the differences between casein, whey and soy vis a vis muscle protein synthesis and the initial peak in plasma amino acids.[61]

4. List some of the benefits of post-workout supplementation found in US Marine Recruits.[59]

Exercise 3

True (A) or False (B)

1. Not consuming anything post-workout has been shown to be an effective strategy in enhancing recovery or promoting gains in LBM.

2. Nutrient timing strategies includes consuming carbohydrate, caffeine and protein at certain times to enhance recovery and/or performance.

3. Consuming caffeine post-workout has been shown to aid in glycogen repletion.

4. Milk based proteins are superior to soy in promoting

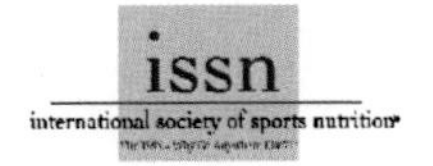

muscle protein synthesis when consumed post-exercise.

5. Consuming a high-glycemic index carbohydrate 10 minutes or less before a prolonged endurance event can help improve performance.

6. The best nutrient timing strategy to combat the detrimental effect of dehydration during a prolonged endurance race is to wait until you are finished to consume water.

7. Consuming a traditional sports drink during exercise lasting > 2 hours can improve performance better than water alone.

8. Post exercise protein supplementation can positively impact health, hydration and tissue soreness.[59]

9. Consuming non-essential amino acids pre-resistance exercise has been shown to promote muscle protein synthesis.

10. Doing 2-a-days (training in the morning and again in the afternoon as seen in American football) would be a circumstance in which consuming a carbohydrate + protein shake immediately post-workout is a smart strategy.

FUN FACT! *John Ivy PhD was a pioneer on the field of carbohydrate metabolism. He conducted some of the original work on the timing of carbohydrate ingestion post-exercise. Folks forget sugar is a damn good ergogenic aid. Dang…where's that Coca-Cola I was drinking…*

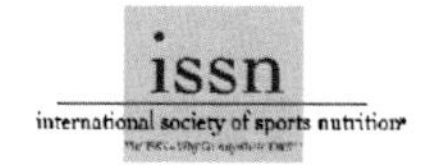

CHAPTER 8 - DIETS AND BODY COMPOSITION

Exercise 1

1. Which of the following contribute the greatest amount with regards to TDEE or total daily energy expenditure?
    a. TEF (thermic effect of food)
    b. RMR (resting metabolic rate)
    c. Exercise
    d. They are all equal in contribution
2. _______________ (NEAT) is the energy expenditure of all physical activities other than volitional sporting-like exercise.[62]
    a. non-energy actual timing
    b. non-exercise activity timing
    c. non-exercise activity thermogenesis
    d. non-exercise activity expenditure
3. The method of body composition that relies on air displacement plethysmography is
    a. Hydrodensitometry
    b. Bod Pod
    c. Magnetic resonance imaging (MRI)
    d. Bioelectrical impedance analysis (BIA)
4. _______________ is a method of body composition that uses measures of body weight, body volume and residual lung volume.
    a. DEXA
    b. BIA
    c. Hydrodensitometry (aka underwater weighing or UWW)
    d. MRI
5. Which of the following body composition techniques utilizes low-dose radiation and can measure bone mineral content?
    a. DEXA
    b. UWW
    c. BIA
    d. All of the above
6. When overweight individuals were put on a isoenergetic low-fat, high carbohydrate diet (HC) versus a high-fat, very-low carbohydrate diet (LC) for 52 weeks, the following was discovered:[63]
    a. The LC group diet promoted greater fat use during submaximal aerobic exercise.

   b. Both groups had similar gains in aerobic capacity.
   c. Both groups had similar gains in strength.
   d. All of the above
7. Increasing protein intake (and thus total energy intake) while keeping exercise energy expenditure the same will likely result in:[13]
   a. An increase in fat mass
   b. An increase in lean body mass
   c. An increase in fat mass and lean body mass
   d. No change in fat mass or lean body mass
8. Which of the following would likely have the greatest thermic effect (isocaloric servings)?
   a. Beans
   b. Steak
   c. Peanut butter
   d. Lard
9. A hot ginger beverage can have the following effect in overweight men:[64]
   a. Enhanced thermogenesis
   b. Reduced feelings of hunger
   c. Increased protein synthesis
   d. A and B are correct
10. In studies that compare low-carbohydrate versus low-fat diets (with protein content the same),
    a. Weight loss tends to be greater with low-fat diets
    b. Weight loss tends to be greater with low-carbohydrate diets
    c. Weight loss is similar
    d. Gains in FFM are greater in the low-fat condition
11. Which of the following are true regarding body composition estimation?
    a. The BIA involves running an electrical current through the body.
    b. DEXA scans involve the exposure of the subject or patient to a low dose of radiation.
    c. The Bod Pod estimates body density via air displacement.
    d. All of the above are true

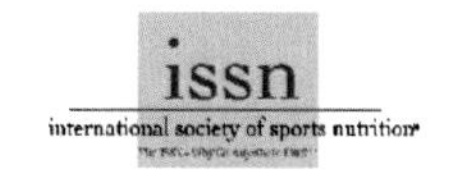

Exercise 2

1. Discuss briefly if consuming a high or low protein diet for ~ 2 months modifies the thermic response to a standard meal.[65]

2. Discuss briefly how meal timing/pattern impacts the TEF.[66]

3. Discuss briefly what happens regarding an isocaloric low-carbohydrate ketogenic diet versus a high carbohydrate diet on changes in body composition.[67]

4. Describe briefly the differences (if any) in dietary protein requirements between young and old individuals.[24]

5. Describe briefly the effects of breakfasts higher in protein on measures of appetite, energy expenditure and fat oxidation.[68]

6. Regarding the most often used measures of body composition in sports science labs (underwater weighing, DEXA, and Bod Pod), which are two- versus three-compartment models?

Exercise 3

True (A) or False (B)

1. In general, diets (hypoenergetic) that are either low-carbohydrate/high fat versus high-carbohydrate/low fat (with equal protein) tend to produce similar results in terms of body weight loss. That is, neither diet is better.

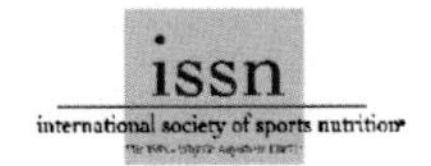

2. In general, the isocaloric substitution of protein for carbohydrate tends to improve body composition (if all else is kept the same).

3. There is ample evidence to suggest that the Mediterranean diet can confer benefits in terms of lowering CVD risk.

4. Protein overfeeding in the absence of other changes has been shown to have a neutral effect on body composition.

5. The prolonged consumption of a high-protein diet does not modify the thermogenic response to a standard meal (i.e., there is not a 'metabolic adaptation' to a high protein diet).[65]

6. A very low-carbohydrate diet is an effective alternative (to other diets such as one that is low in fat) in improving exercise capacity in overweight and obese adults.[63]

7. There is robust evidence to show that a ketogenic diet has a performance-enhancing effect in running races of 10k to a half-marathon.

8. An irregular meal frequency has been shown to have a negative effect by decreasing the thermic effect of food.[66]

9. During a marked energy deficit, consumption of a diet containing 2.4 g/kg/d of protein was more effective than a diet of 1.2 g/kg/d (of protein) in promoting increases in LBM and losses of fat mass in conjunction with a high volume of resistance and anaerobic exercise.[69]

10. Increased soy protein intake attenuated gains in muscle strength during resistance training in older adults compared with increased intake of dairy protein.[70]

FUN FACT! *Work from James Hill PhD suggests that NEAT can vary substantially between individuals by as much as 2000 kcal/d. Whoa. You can eat a lot of cheeseburgers if you move that much.*

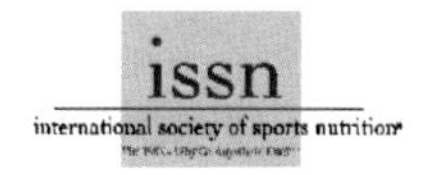

CHAPTER 9 – FUNCTIONAL FOODS

1. Regular coffee consumption is associated with[71]
    a. Reduced mortality
    b. Reduced heart disease
    c. Reduced diabetes
    d. All of the above
2. Observational data suggest that heavy coffee consumption[72]
    a. May decrease the risk of stroke
    b. May increase the risk of stroke
    c. May increase the risk of type II diabetes
    d. May decrease the risk of pancreatic cancer
3. The primary active ingredient in energy drinks (e.g., Red Bull) is
    a. Taurine
    b. Caffeine
    c. Sugar
    d. Both B and C
4. Studies on green tea extract regarding performance enhancement have generally shown
    a. A significant performance enhancement effect
    b. No effect
    c. A significant detriment to performance
    d. A significant improvement in strength only
5. Limited evidence suggests that tart cherry juice
    a. May lessen muscle damage
    b. May improve recovery
    c. May lower post-exercise pain
    d. All of the above
6. Acute beetroot juice supplementation may[73]
    a. Attenuate muscle soreness
    b. Increase muscle soreness
    c. Be pro-inflammatory
    d. None of the above
7. A single dose of beetroot juice ____________ during submaximal exercise and __________ time trial performance[74] of trained cyclists in normobaric hypoxia.
    a. Lowers oxygen uptake, enhances
    b. Increases oxygen uptake, worsens
    c. Lowers oxygen uptake, worsens
    d. Increases oxygen uptake, enhances
8. Which of the following foods have scientific data to support their use as an ergogenic aid?

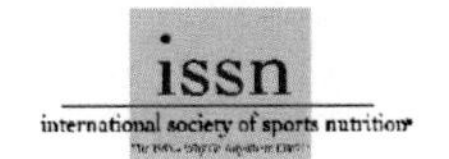

   a. Apples
   b. White bread
   c. Broccoli
   d. Chocolate milk
9. In comparison to an isocaloric carbohydrate drink, the consumption of fat-free milk immediately after and then one-hour post-exercise in young women showed that[75]
   a. Milk produced better gains in FFM
   b. Milk produced better gains in strength
   c. Milk produced fat mass loss
   d. All of the above
10. Chronic dark chocolate supplementation[76]
   a. May enhance time trial performance
   b. Reduces the oxygen cost of moderate intensity exercise
   c. Is an effective ergogenic aid for short-duration moderate intensity exercise
   d. All of the above

Exercise 2

1. Describe briefly the basic theory behind the possible ergogenic effect of beetroot juice.[74]

2. Describe briefly the role of whole grain intake regarding mortality, CVD, CHD, stroke and diabetes based on this observational study.[77]

3. Describe briefly the effects of fish oil plus aerobic exercise on CVD risk factors and body composition.[78]

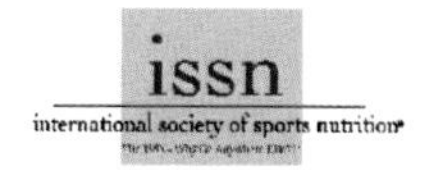

4. Describe briefly the effect of coffee consumption on overall and cause-specific mortality.[71]

5. Describe briefly the effects of beer drinking vis a vis hydration.[79]

Exercise 3

True (A) or False (B)

1. Regular consumption of coffee has been shown to decrease the risk of type II diabetes.

2. Moderate beer intake has no harmful effects on markers of hydration post-exercise.

3. Fiber from whole grains (but not refined grains) is associated with a drop in all-cause mortality.

4. The consumption of milk post-exercise has been shown to be an effective choice for re-hydration.

5. Heavy coffee consumption is associated with a drop in stroke prevalence.[72]

6. Observational data suggests that the consumption of chocolate is associated with a lower risk of coronary heart disease.[80]

7. There is evidence to suggest that the regular consumption of green tea may reduce the risk of all-cause mortality.[81]

8. There is robust evidence via randomized controlled trials which demonstrate that consuming whole grains on a regular basis improves gains in lean body mass.

9. The acute consumption of beetroot juice has been shown

to enhance performance in aerobic events; however, not all studies show an ergogenic effect.[82, 83]

10. The regular consumption of dairy protein (e.g., milk) is associated with gains in fat mass.

FUN FACT! *Work by Richardson and Clarke (2016) showed that coffee and decaf-coffee with added caffeine can improve resistance exercise performance. Yes sir. Drink java and lift heavy stuff.*

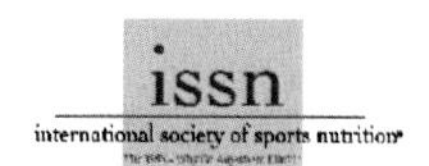

CHAPTER 10 – ERGOGENIC SPORTS SUPPLEMENTS

Exercise 1

1. With regards to probiotics, which of the following are true?[84, 85]
    a. Are live microorganisms
    b. May increase running time to fatigue in the heat
    c. May impact mood
    d. All of the above
2. Chronic betaine supplementation may[86]
    a. Increase type IIX muscle fiber size
    b. Increase capillary density
    c. Increase total volume of exercise performed
    d. All of the above
3. Glycerol-containing beverages create an osmotic gradient in the circulation favoring fluid __________, thereby facilitating ______________ and protecting against dehydration.[87]
    a. Retention, hyperhydration
    b. Loss, hyperhydration
    c. Retention, dehydration
    d. None of the above
4. Phosphatidic acid ingestion (750 mg/d), combined with a 4-day per week resistance training program for 2 months in young, resistance-trained individuals may cause the following:[88]
    a. Strength improvement
    b. Lean tissue enhancement
    c. Gain in body fat
    d. Only A and B are correct
5. There is evidence to suggest that supplementing with L-glutamine at a dose of 0.3 g/kg once per day over 72 hours post-eccentric exercise[89]
    a. Lowers muscle soreness
    b. Promotes a faster recovery of peak torque
    c. Enhances the removal of lactate
    d. Both A and B are correct
6. Consuming alpha glycerylphosphorylcholine (alpha-GPC) at a dose of _______ can enhance lower body force production after _________ days of supplementation.[90]
    a. 600 mg/d, 6 days
    b. 6 g/d, 6 days
    c. 6 g/d, 60 days

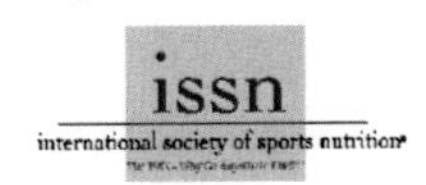

   d. Has no ergogenic effect
7. Beta-hydroxy-methyl-butyrate (HMB)
   a. May have an anti-catabolic effect
   b. Has been shown to preferentially increase type IIX muscle fiber size
   c. Is a downstream metabolite of isoleucine
   d. Two of the above are correct
8. Phosphatidylserine administration at a dose of ______ for 10 days may ________________.[91]
   a. 750 mg/d, improve time to exhaustion
   b. 7 g/d, improve time to exhaustion
   c. 7 mg/d, improve time to exhaustion
   d. 10 g/d, improve muscular strength
9. The ingestion of the ___________ dipeptide at either the low or high dose significantly improved time to exhaustion during high-intensity exercise compared to a no-hydration trial.[92]
   a. Alanine-glutamine
   b. Alanine-leucine
   c. Leucine-glutamine
   d. Glycine-glutamine
10. There is evidence that suggests arachidonic acid supplementation may _____________ in trained men.[93]
   a. Enhance lean body mass and upper body strength
   b. Enhance $maxVO_2$
   c. Decrease bone mineral density
   d. None of the above

Exercise 2

List a potential ergogenic benefit of the following supplements:

1. Probiotics

2. Betaine

3. Glycerol

4. Phosphatidic acid

5. Glutamine

6. HMB

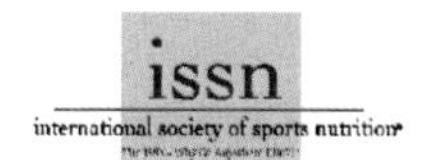

7. L-alanyl-L-glutamine
8. Alpha-GPC
9. Arachidonic acid

Exercise 3

True (A) or False (B)

1. There is evidence to suggest that probiotic supplementation can positively affect mood and mental health.[94]
2. L-glutamine is the most abundant amino acid in the body.
3. The activation of mTOR by resistance training depends on the synthesis of phosphatidic acid.
4. In general, studies have shown that D-ribose supplementation confers little to no performance-enhancing effect on healthy trained and untrained populations.
5. The acute consumption of Alpha-GPC will elevate plasma choline levels.
6. HMB has been shown in various clinical trials to promote gains in LBM with 3 g daily as an efficacious dose.
7. There is evidence to suggest that glycerol-induced hyperhydration may improve overall exercise performance and time to exhaustion.
8. Probiotics have been shown to reduce upper respiratory tract infections as well as gastrointestinal distress.
9. There is evidence to suggest that quercetin my promote mitochondrial biogenesis.
10. Phosphatidylserine is a phospholipid found in cell membranes of most animals and plants.

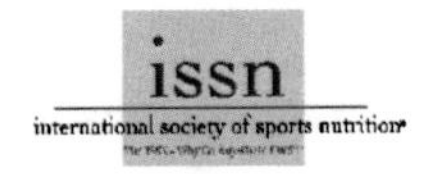

CHAPTER 11 – BETA-ALANINE[95]

Exercise 1

1. Four weeks of beta-alanine supplementation ___________significantly augments muscle carnosine concentrations, thereby acting as an intracellular pH buffer.
    a. 4-6 mg daily
    b. 0.4-0.6 grams daily
    c. 4-6 grams daily
    d. 40-60 mg daily
2. Beta-alanine is a __________ amino acid that is produced endogenously in the ________.
    a. Non-essential, bone marrow
    b. Essential, liver
    c. Essential, adrenal medulla
    d. Non-essential, liver
3. Carnosine is a naturally occurring dipeptide with numerous potential physiological functions and is formed by combining its constituent amino acids, _______ and beta-alanine, with the assistance of the enzyme carnosine synthetase.
    a. L-arginine
    b. L-leucine
    c. L-histidine
    d. None of the above
4. In general, current studies suggest that beta-alanine supplementation can improve exercise capacity in tasks lasting
    a. 6-30 seconds
    b. 1-4 minutes
    c. 1-40 minutes
    d. 1-10 seconds
5. The most widely known side effect of beta-alanine supplementation is
    a. Diuresis
    b. Increased plasma lactate
    c. Paraesthesia
    d. All of the above
6. Research has demonstrated _________ of beta-alanine supplementation on TTE in exercise tests over 4 min in duration.

   a. No benefit
   b. A modest benefit
   c. A slight detriment
   d. A enormous benefit
7. The combination of HIIT (high intensity interval training) and beta-alanine supplementation[96]
   a. May enhance HIIT performance
   b. May further increase LBM
   c. May improve endurance
   d. All of the above
8. The median effect of beta-alanine supplementation (2.85% improvement) occurs when the median total of _____ of beta-alanine in consumed.
   a. 17.9 grams
   b. 179 mg
   c. 179 grams
   d. 1,079 grams
9. While cross-sectional studies have shown ______ baseline carnosine contents in the *gastrocnemius* muscle of sprinters and resistance-trained athletes versus their untrained counterparts, beta-alanine supplementation has also been shown to increase muscle carnosine in ______________.
   a. Lower, both trained and untrained populations.
   b. Higher, both trained and untrained populations.
   c. Higher, in trained but not in untrained populations.
   d. Lower, in trained populations primarily.
10. __________, the enzyme that catalyzes the breakdown of carnosine, is present in serum and various tissues in humans.
   a. Phosphofructokinase
   b. Carnosinase
   c. Hexokinase
   d. Creatine Kinase

Exercise 2

1. Describe the basic mechanism(s) in which beta-alanine supplementation can provide an ergogenic effect.

2. How long does it take to observe a performance-enhancing effect of beta-alanine supplementation?

3. What is carnosine?

4. Approximately what is the *total* dose needed to observe an ergogenic effect?

5. Describe the effects of combining beta-alanine and sodium bicarbonate on 2000 meter rowing performance.[97]

6. Describe how beta-alanine supplementation helps (or not) varying distances in cycling.[98]

7. Is there an ergogenic effect of beta-alanine supplementation in combat soliders?[99]

Exercise 3

True (A) or False (B)[95]

1. Four weeks of beta-alanine supplementation (4-6 g daily) significantly augments muscle carnosine concentrations.

2. Beta-alanine supplementation currently appears to be safe in healthy populations at recommended doses.

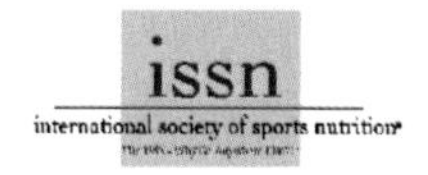

3. The only reported side effect is paraesthesia (i.e., tingling), but studies indicate this can be attenuated by using divided lower doses (1.6 g).

4. Daily supplementation with 4 to 6 g of beta-alanine for at least 2 to 4 weeks has been shown to improve exercise performance.

5. Beta-alanine is a non-essential amino acid.

6. Beta-alanine would be a great ergogenic aid for the 400m race in track and field.

7. Beta-alanine improves tactical performance in combat soldiers.

8. Beta-alanine exerts its best ergogenic effects in events lasting 1-4 minutes.

9. Beta-alanine combines with histidine to form carnosine.

10. Beta-alanine has been identified as the rate-limiting precursor to carnosine synthesis.

FUN FACT! *If you want to learn the latest sports nutrition science, the best resources include: (1) peer-reviewed science journals (e.g., JISSN, IJSNEM, AJCN, JSCR, etc.), (2) science conferences (e.g., ISSN, NSCA, etc.) and (3) networking with scientists (who do the research) and practitioners who implement the science.*

Relying on third-party websites (e.g., WebMD, Wikipedia, etc.) may result in a statistically significant decrease [$p<0.05$] in your sports nutrition science IQ. And beware of the Twitter and Facebook experts who earned their PhDs from the University of Google. They are so certain of their pre-conceived beliefs that you could pi$$ on their feet and they'd think it's raining. So buyer beware.

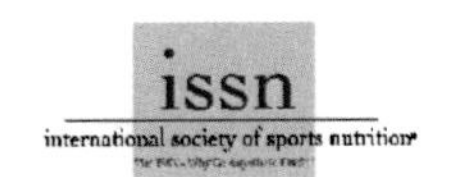

Answer Key

Chapter 1 – Bioenergetics and Skeletal Muscle

Exercise 1

1. D
2. A
3. A
4. A
5. A
6. C
7. C
8. B
9. C
10. C

Exercise 2

1. In general, there is a continuum with regards to characteristics of Type I, IIA and IIX fibers. Mitochondrial volume/density – highest in type I, then type IIA, and lastly type IIX. Capillary density – highest in type I, then type IIA, and lastly type IIX. Contractile speed – fastest in type IIX, then IIA and then I. Refer to any exercise physiology text for more information.
2. High jump, javelin, shot put
3. 400 meter dash, wrestling, MMA
4. Any distance in running races from the 1500 or longer (ex. 1500m, 3000m SC, 5k, 10k, half-marathon etc.)
5. Satellite cells functions include: repair of damaged skeletal muscle fibers as well as promotion of hypertrophy and in some instances, hyperplasia.

Exercise 3

1. B
2. B
3. B
4. A
5. A
6. B
7. A
8. B

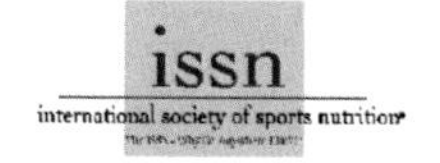

9. A
10. B

Exercise 4

1. A
2. B
3. A
4. A
5. A
6. A
7. A
8. A
9. A
10. A

Chapter 2 – Protein and Amino Acids

Exercise 1

1. B
2. D
3. B
4. C
5. D
6. D
7. C
8. D
9. D
10. B

Exercise 2

1. Ingestion 40 g of whey protein following whole body resistance training promotes a greater MPS response than 20 g in young trained men.
2. A higher protein diet promotes an increase in LBM and drop in fat mass when combined with a traditional bodybuilding training routine. Note: the lower protein group increased LBM but had no fat mass change.
3. Protein spread theory – there must be a sufficient difference in g/kg/d of protein intake between groups to get changes in LBM and/or strength. Protein change

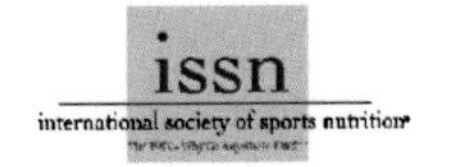

theory – there must be a sufficient change from baseline in protein intake to see changes in LBM and/or strength.

4. Older (~71 yr.) individuals are less sensitive to protein intake vis a vis MPS than young individuals (~22 yr.).
5. Leucine
6. Remember PVT TIM HALL as your mnemonic device: Phenylalanine, threonine, tryptophan, isoleucine, methionine, histidine*, (arginine is conditionally essential), lysine, leucine. (*histidine is produced in adequate amounts in adults; but is essential in children).

Exercise 3

1. A
2. A
3. A
4. A
5. B
6. A
7. A
8. B
9. A
10. A

Chapter 3 - Carbohydrate

Exercise 1

1. D
2. A
3. D
4. A
5. A
6. B
7. B
8. C
9. A
10. D

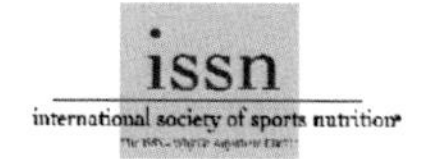

Exercise 2

1. Deplete skeletal muscle glycogen over a 3 day period via exhaustive exercise and by eating a lower carb diet (<5% of dietary energy). Subsequently, perform 3 days of exhaustive exercise followed by a high-carb diet (>90% of dietary energy).
2. In general, carb intake pre and during a race or game will improve performance.
3. According to Jeukendrup, studies have shown that oral carbohydrate mouth rinses may improve performance roughly 2% and 3% during exercise lasting approximately 1 hour (compared to a placebo).
4. The classic advice has been to consume 30-60 g per hour; however, newer work shows that oxidation rates can reach much higher values (up to 105 g/h) when multiple transportable carbohydrates are ingested (i.e. glucose:fructose).
5. Myth – that you shouldn't consume carbohydrate in the hour pre-exercise due to rebound hypoglycemia. Though symptoms of hypoglycemia may occur, it does not seem to affect performance.

Exercise 3

1. ~60 grams per hour
2. ~90 grams per hour

Exercise 4

1. A
2. A
3. A
4. B
5. A

Chapter 4 - Fat

Exercise 1

1. C
2. A
3. C

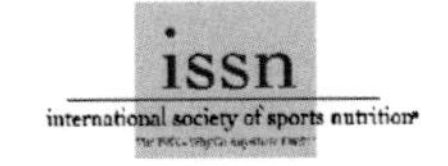

4. A
5. A
6. D
7. D
8. A
9. C
10. D

Exercise 2

1. Mean MFO = 0.59 g/min; MFO was higher in females than males when expressed per unit FFM (11 vs. 10 mg/kg/min). Soccer players were the highest in this group (10.8 mg/kg/min); American football players were lowest (9.2 mg/kg/min).
2. Fat oxidation was found to be higher during rowing compared to cycling across a range of exercise intensities matched for energy expenditure. This may be a consequence of larger muscle mass recruited during rowing.
3. Fish oil consumption resulted in: lower triglycerides, increased energy expenditure during exercise, increased LBM.
4. Inconsistent results in terms of weight loss. Some possible adverse effects on glucose metabolism and lipid profile.
5. There is no difference in body composition whether one is fed or fasted pre-cardio exercise.

Exercise 3

1. A
2. A
3. A
4. A
5. B
6. A
7. A
8. A
9. A
10. A

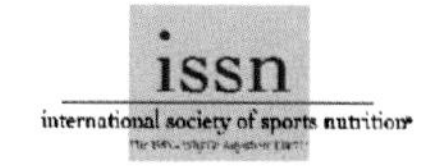

Chapter 5 - Creatine

Exercise 1

1. B
2. A
3. B
4. D
5. C
6. B
7. B
8. D
9. C
10. B

Exercise 2

1. Typically it involves consuming 20g/d of creatine (in divided doses) for ~ a week.
2. Methionine, arginine, and glycine
3. Creatine has a more profound effect on vegans in terms of memory enhancement.
4. Creatine can actually augment skeletal muscle glycogen repletion when combined with carbohydrate.
5. Shot put, discus, hammer, high jump, long jump, triple jump, pole vault etc.
6. When compared to creatine monohydrate, creatine ethyl ester was not as effective at increasing serum and muscle creatine levels or in improving body composition, muscle mass, strength, and power.
7. Creatine supplementation increases type I, IIA and IIX myosin heavy chain mRNA expression as well as MHC protein.
8. Creatine is a benefit to those with certain types of muscular dystrophy and idiopathic inflammatory myopathies.
9. Changes in muscle mass were similar in older adults. It did not matter if creatine was ingested pre or post exercise.

Exercise 3

1. B
2. B
3. A

4. B
5. A
6. A
7. A
8. A
9. A
10. A

Chapter 6 - Caffeine

Exercise 1

1. C
2. B
3. B
4. D
5. D
6. D
7. D
8. D
9. B
10. A

Exercise 2

1. Individuals who are homozygous for the A allele of this polymorphism (CYP1A2 gene) respond best to caffeine.
2. While 1 mg/kg had no effect, 3 mg/kg did improve half-squat and bench press maximal power.
3. Supplementation with 100 mg of *p*-synephrine alone and in combination with 100 mg of caffeine significantly augmented resistance exercise performance.
4. Distance running (numerous events), powerlifting, soccer, rugby, rowing, etc. (note: caffeine can help virtually all types of exercise).
5. Caffeine-naïve individuals respond better than those who are regular consumers.
6. Improved CNS alertness, enhanced lipolysis, increased pain threshold, enhanced thermic effect etc.
7. ~3-6 mg/kg
8. Headaches, dizziness, anxiety, restlessness, insomnia, etc.
9. Caffeine and caffeinated coffee can enhance performance.

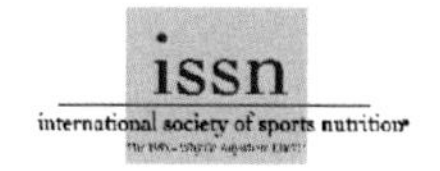

Exercise 3

1. A
2. A
3. A
4. A
5. A
6. A
7. B
8. A
9. A
10. A

Chapter 7 – Nutrient Timing

Exercise 1

1. B
2. A
3. A
4. D
5. D
6. D
7. C
8. A
9. A
10. C

Exercise 2

1. Performing 2-a-days (ex. American football practice), endurance exercise lasting 90 minutes or longer, multiple bouts of exercise or competition over several days, high volume resistance training, etc.
2. Four feedings of 20 grams of whey protein consumed ever 3 hours (intermediate) was better than Pulse feeding (8 feedings of 10 grams every 1.5 hours) and Bolus feeding (2 feedings of 40 grams every 6 hours) in terms of stimulating MPS. (Note: total protein intake is 80 grams). In summary: 4 x 20g > 8 x 10g or 2 x 40g
3. In terms of reaching peak time to muscle protein synthesis, whey protein was fastest followed by milk proteins and lastly casein. Also milk based proteins are more effective than soy vis a vis protein synthesis.

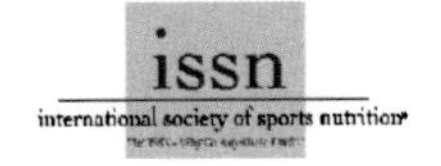

4. Compared with placebo and control groups, the protein-supplemented group had an average of 33% fewer total medical visits, 28% fewer visits due to bacterial/viral infections, 37% fewer visits due to muscle/joint problems, and 83% fewer visits due to heat exhaustion.

Exercise 3

1. B
2. A
3. A
4. A
5. A
6. B
7. A
8. A
9. B
10. A

Chapter 8 – Diets and Body Composition

Exercise 1

1. B
2. C
3. B
4. C
5. A
6. D
7. D
8. B
9. D
10. C
11. D

Exercise 2

1. There is no metabolic adaptation to consuming a high protein diet.
2. There is a reduced TEF with an irregular (vs. regular) meal pattern.
3. An isocaloric ketogenic diet was not accompanied by an increased body fat loss.

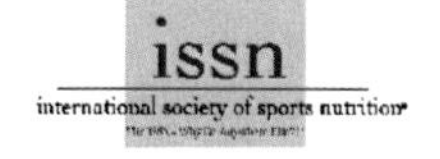

4. Healthy older men (~71 yr.) are less sensitive to low protein intakes and require a greater relative protein intake, in a single meal, than young men (~22 yr.) to maximally stimulate postprandial rates of MPS.
5. A protein-based breakfast increases postprandial EE and fat oxidation, reduces hunger, and increases satiety when compared with a carbohydrate-based breakfast.
6. 2-compartment models (fat and lean body mass) – underwater weighing, Bod Pod. 3-compartment model – DEXA (fat, bone, and bone-free lean tissue mass)

Exercise 3

1. A
2. A
3. A
4. A
5. A
6. A
7. B
8. A
9. A
10. A

Chapter 9 – Functional Foods

Exercise 1

1. D
2. A
3. D
4. B
5. D
6. A
7. A
8. D
9. D
10. D

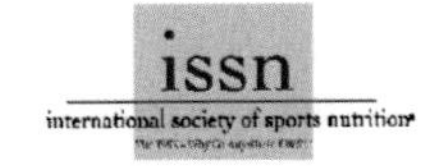

Exercise 2

1. Consuming beetroot juice may increase nitric oxide availability. This may improve performance by lowering the oxygen cost of exercise.
2. Observational data suggest that there is an inverse relationship between whole grain consumption and risk of mortality from CVD and CHD.
3. Fish oil plus exercise may reduce body fat levels and decrease CVD risk.
4. Cohort data suggest that drinking coffee lowers the risk of heart disease, diabetes, chronic respirator diseases etc.
5. After exercise and subsequent dehydration, a moderate bee intake has no deleterious effects on markers of hydration in active individuals.

Exercise 3

1. A
2. A
3. A
4. A
5. A
6. A
7. A
8. B
9. A
10. B

Chapter 10 – Ergogenic Sports Supplements

Exercise 1

1. D
2. C
3. A
4. D
5. D
6. A
7. D
8. A
9. A
10. A

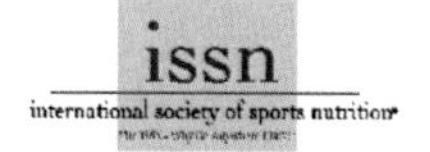

Exercise 2

1. Probiotics – may reduce indices of muscle damage, improve recovery. May also benefit the immune system, mood, mental health and perhaps body composition in the overweight
2. Betaine - Limited evidence to show it may improve muscle endurance, power and force; reduce subjective measures of fatigue etc.
3. Glycerol – may aid in hydration
4. Phosphatidic acid – may benefit strength and LBM gains
5. Glutamine – lower risk of URTI following severe exercise; potentially less muscle soreness post-eccentric exercise
6. HMB – anti-catabolic effect, may enhance LBM gains, lessens muscle loss during an energy deficit
7. L-alanyl-l-glutamine – may improve time to exhaustion during mild hydration stress
8. Alpha-GPC – may improve lower body force production
9. Arachidonic acid – may improve LBM and strength

Exercise 3

1. A
2. A
3. A
4. A
5. A
6. A
7. A
8. A
9. A
10. A

Chapter 11 – Beta-Alanine

Exercise 1

1. C
2. D
3. C
4. B
5. C
6. B

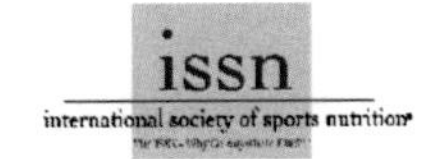

7. D
8. C
9. B
10. B

Exercise 2

1. By forming carnosine (via beta-alanine + histidine), this aids performance vis a vis an intramuscular buffer
2. Approximately 2-4 weeks (depending on the dose)
3. Carnosine is a dipeptide in skeletal muscle. Its acts as an intramuscular buffer.
4. 179 grams
5. The addition of sodium bicarbonate to chronic beta-alanine supplementation may further enhance rowing performance
6. In highly trained cyclists, beta-alanine helps in a 4-km time trial but not in a 1 or 10-km time trial
7. May enhance target engagement speed and marksmanship in soldiers

Exercise 3

1. A
2. A
3. A
4. A
5. A
6. A
7. A
8. A
9. A
10. A

ABOUT THE AUTHOR

Jose Antonio, Ph.D. FISSN FNSCA CSCS is the CEO and co-founder of the **International Society of Sports Nutrition** (www.issn.net). Dr. Antonio is an Associate Professor of Exercise and Sports Science at Nova Southeastern University in beautiful South Florida. He has two offices. One on campus (no window view, so sad) and one on the ocean. In his spare time, he watches his wife and daughters race (distance running, duathlons, track and field). When he's not writing, he's usually watching TV (MMA and football [not soccer]), paddling around South Florida, or overeating at a local sushi dive. On a semi-serious note, he earned his PhD and completed a post-doctoral research fellowship at the *University of Texas Southwestern Medical Center* and has written over a dozen books and countless articles – enough to cure anyone's insomnia. Lastly, his coffee and rice addiction will never be cured. Thank you.
Twitter @JoseAntonioPhD

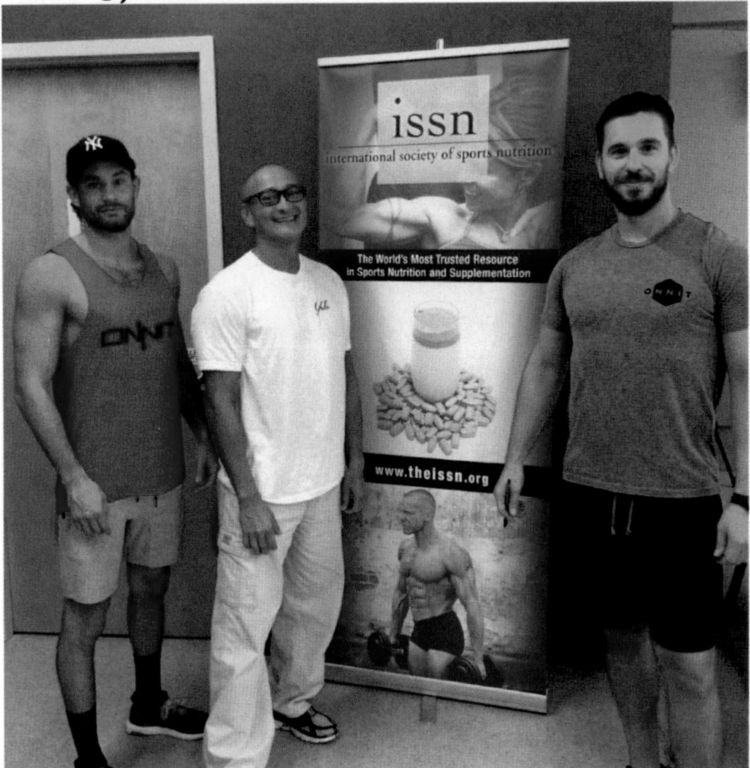

L-R: **Chris Algieri CISSN**, yours truly, and **Corey Peacock PhD CISSN** – After a day of data collection for a study on the ***ACTN3 genotype***.

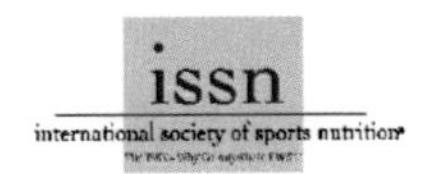

REFERENCES

1. Antonio J and International Society of Sport Nutrition.: Essentials of sports nutrition and supplements. Totowa, NJ: Humana Press; 2008(Series Editor)
2. Greenwood M, Kalman D, and Antonio J: Nutritional supplements in sports and exercise. Totowa, N.J.: Humana Press; 2008(Series Editor)
3. Antonio J and Gonyea WJ: Skeletal muscle fiber hyperplasia. Med Sci Sports Exerc 1993, 25:1333-45.
4. Schiaffino S and Reggiani C: Myosin isoforms in mammalian skeletal muscle. J Appl Physiol (1985) 1994, 77:493-501.
5. A. Smith-Ryan & J Antonio, 2013. Sports Nutrition & Performance Enhancing Supplements. Linus Books.
6. Antonio J, Ellerbroek A, Silver T, et al.: The effects of a high protein diet on indices of health and body composition--a crossover trial in resistance-trained men. J Int Soc Sports Nutr 2016, 13:3.
7. Mobley CB, Hornberger TA, Fox CD, et al.: Effects of oral phosphatidic acid feeding with or without whey protein on muscle protein synthesis and anabolic signaling in rodent skeletal muscle. J Int Soc Sports Nutr 2015, 12:32.
8. Hulmi JJ, Laakso M, Mero AA, et al.: The effects of whey protein with or without carbohydrates on resistance training adaptations. J Int Soc Sports Nutr 2015, 12:48.
9. Babault N, Paizis C, Deley G, et al.: Pea proteins oral supplementation promotes muscle thickness gains during resistance training: A double-blind, randomized, placebo-controlled clinical trial vs. Whey protein. J Int Soc Sports Nutr 2015, 12:3.
10. Antonio J, Ellerbroek A, Silver T, et al.: A high protein diet (3.4 g/kg/d) combined with a heavy resistance training program improves body composition in healthy trained men and women--a follow-up investigation. J Int Soc Sports Nutr 2015, 12:39.
11. Wang X, Niu C, Lu J, et al.: Hydrolyzed protein supplementation improves protein content and

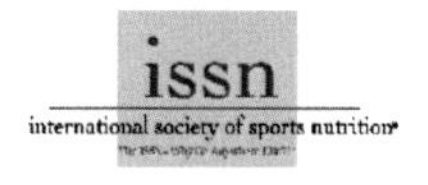

peroxidation of skeletal muscle by adjusting the plasma amino acid spectrums in rats after exhaustive swimming exercise: A pilot study. J Int Soc Sports Nutr 2014, 11:5.

12. Babault N, Deley G, Le Ruyet P, et al.: Effects of soluble milk protein or casein supplementation on muscle fatigue following resistance training program: A randomized, double-blind, and placebo-controlled study. J Int Soc Sports Nutr 2014, 11:36.
13. Antonio J, Peacock CA, Ellerbroek A, et al.: The effects of consuming a high protein diet (4.4 g/kg/d) on body composition in resistance-trained individuals. J Int Soc Sports Nutr 2014, 11:19.
14. Schoenfeld BJ, Aragon AA, and Krieger JW: The effect of protein timing on muscle strength and hypertrophy: A meta-analysis. J Int Soc Sports Nutr 2013, 10:53.
15. Stark M, Lukaszuk J, Prawitz A, et al.: Protein timing and its effects on muscular hypertrophy and strength in individuals engaged in weight-training. J Int Soc Sports Nutr 2012, 9:54.
16. Bosse JD and Dixon BM: Dietary protein to maximize resistance training: A review and examination of protein spread and change theories. J Int Soc Sports Nutr 2012, 9:42.
17. Kim H, Lee S, and Choue R: Metabolic responses to high protein diet in korean elite bodybuilders with high-intensity resistance exercise. J Int Soc Sports Nutr 2011, 8:10.
18. Cooke MB, Rybalka E, Stathis CG, et al.: Whey protein isolate attenuates strength decline after eccentrically-induced muscle damage in healthy individuals. J Int Soc Sports Nutr 2010, 7:30.
19. Lowery LM and Devia L: Dietary protein safety and resistance exercise: What do we really know? J Int Soc Sports Nutr 2009, 6:3.
20. Campbell B, Kreider RB, Ziegenfuss T, et al.: International society of sports nutrition position stand: Protein and exercise. J Int Soc Sports Nutr 2007, 4:8.

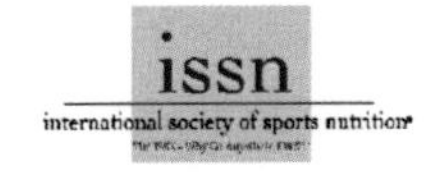

21. Palop Montoro MV, Parraga Montilla JA, Lozano Aguilera E, et al.: [sarcopenia intervention with progressive resistance training and protein nutritional supplements]. Nutr Hosp 2015, 31:1481-90.
22. Witard OC, Wardle SL, Macnaughton LS, et al.: Protein considerations for optimising skeletal muscle mass in healthy young and older adults. Nutrients 2016, 8:181.
23. Macnaughton LS, Wardle SL, Witard OC, et al.: The response of muscle protein synthesis following whole-body resistance exercise is greater following 40 g than 20 g of ingested whey protein. Physiol Rep 2016, 4.
24. Moore DR, Churchward-Venne TA, Witard O, et al.: Protein ingestion to stimulate myofibrillar protein synthesis requires greater relative protein intakes in healthy older versus younger men. J Gerontol A Biol Sci Med Sci 2015, 70:57-62.
25. Baker LB, Rollo I, Stein KW, et al.: Acute effects of carbohydrate supplementation on intermittent sports performance. Nutrients 2015, 7:5733-63.
26. Jeukendrup AE: Oral carbohydrate rinse: Placebo or beneficial? Curr Sports Med Rep 2013, 12:222-7.
27. Jeukendrup A: The new carbohydrate intake recommendations. Nestle Nutr Inst Workshop Ser 2013, 75:63-71.
28. Jeukendrup AE and Killer SC: The myths surrounding pre-exercise carbohydrate feeding. Ann Nutr Metab 2010, 57 Suppl 2:18-25.
29. Jeukendrup A: A step towards personalized sports nutrition: Carbohydrate intake during exercise. Sports Med 2014, 44 Suppl 1:S25-33.
30. Randell RK, Rollo I, Roberts TJ, et al.: Maximal fat oxidation rates in an athletic population. Med Sci Sports Exerc 2016.
31. Egan B, Ashley DT, Kennedy E, et al.: Higher rate of fat oxidation during rowing compared with cycling ergometer exercise across a range of exercise intensities. Scand J Med Sci Sports 2016, 26:630-7.

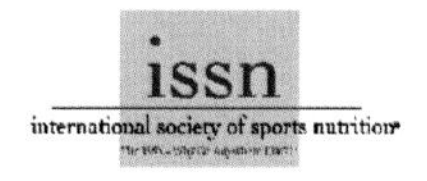

32. Logan SL and Spriet LL: Omega-3 fatty acid supplementation for 12 weeks increases resting and exercise metabolic rate in healthy community-dwelling older females. PLoS One 2015, 10:e0144828.
33. Lehnen TE, da Silva MR, Camacho A, et al.: A review on effects of conjugated linoleic fatty acid (cla) upon body composition and energetic metabolism. J Int Soc Sports Nutr 2015, 12:36.
34. Benjamin S, Prakasan P, Sreedharan S, et al.: Pros and cons of cla consumption: An insight from clinical evidences. Nutr Metab (Lond) 2015, 12:4.
35. Schoenfeld BJ, Aragon AA, Wilborn CD, et al.: Body composition changes associated with fasted versus non-fasted aerobic exercise. J Int Soc Sports Nutr 2014, 11:54.
36. Buford TW, Kreider RB, Stout JR, et al.: International society of sports nutrition position stand: Creatine supplementation and exercise. J Int Soc Sports Nutr 2007, 4:6.
37. Antonio J and Ciccone V: The effects of pre versus post workout supplementation of creatine monohydrate on body composition and strength. Journal of the International Society of Sports Nutrition 2013, 10:36.
38. Lugaresi R, Leme M, de Salles Painelli V, et al.: Does long-term creatine supplementation impair kidney function in resistance-trained individuals consuming a high-protein diet? J Int Soc Sports Nutr 2013, 10:26.
39. Claudino JG, Mezencio B, Amaral S, et al.: Creatine monohydrate supplementation on lower-limb muscle power in brazilian elite soccer players. Journal of the International Society of Sports Nutrition 2014, 11:32.
40. Joy JM, Lowery RP, Falcone PH, et al.: 28 days of creatine nitrate supplementation is apparently safe in healthy individuals. Journal of the International Society of Sports Nutrition 2014, 11:60.
41. Galvan E, Walker DK, Simbo SY, et al.: Acute and chronic safety and efficacy of dose dependent creatine nitrate supplementation and exercise

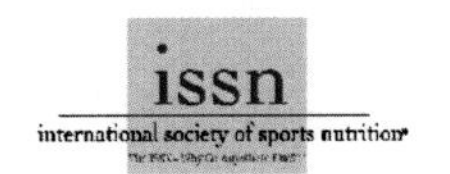

performance. J Int Soc Sports Nutr 2016, 13:12.
42. Kreider R: Sports applications of creatine. In Essentials of sports nutrition and supplements. Edited by Douglas Kalman JA, Jeffrey Stout, Mike Greenwood, Darryn Willoughby, Greg Haff. Totowa, NJ: Humana Press; 2008.
43. McCall W and Persky AM: Pharmacokinetics of creatine. In Creatine and creatine kinase in health and disease. Volume 46. Edited by Salomons GS and Wyss M: Springer Netherlands; 2008:262-273.
44. NELSON AG, ARNALL DA, KOKKONEN J, et al.: Muscle glycogen supercompensation is enhanced by prior creatine supplementation. Medicine & Science in Sports & Exercise 2001, 33:1096-1100.
45. van Loon LJC, Murphy R, Oosterlaar AM, et al.: Creatine supplementation increases glycogen storage but not glut-4 expression in human skeletal muscle. Clinical science 2004, 106:99-106.
46. Benton D and Donohoe R: The influence of creatine supplementation on the cognitive functioning of vegetarians and omnivores. The British journal of nutrition 2011, 105:1100-5.
47. Roberts PA, Fox J, Peirce N, et al.: Creatine ingestion augments dietary carbohydrate mediated muscle glycogen supercompensation during the initial 24 h of recovery following prolonged exhaustive exercise in humans. Amino acids 2016, 48:1831-42.
48. Spillane M, Schoch R, Cooke M, et al.: The effects of creatine ethyl ester supplementation combined with heavy resistance training on body composition, muscle performance, and serum and muscle creatine levels. J Int Soc Sports Nutr 2009, 6:6.
49. Willoughby DS and Rosene J: Effects of oral creatine and resistance training on myosin heavy chain expression. Med Sci Sports Exerc 2001, 33:1674-81.
50. Kley RA, Tarnopolsky MA, and Vorgerd M: Creatine for treating muscle disorders. Cochrane Database Syst Rev 2013:CD004760.
51. Candow DG, Zello GA, Ling B, et al.: Comparison of creatine supplementation before versus after

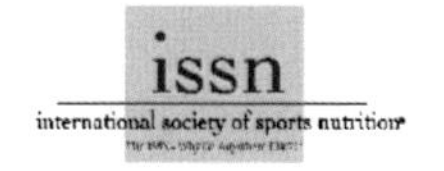

supervised resistance training in healthy older adults. Res Sports Med 2014, 22:61-74.
52. Goldstein ER, Ziegenfuss T, Kalman D, et al.: International society of sports nutrition position stand: Caffeine and performance. J Int Soc Sports Nutr 2010, 7:5.
53. Womack CJ, Saunders MJ, Bechtel MK, et al.: The influence of a cyp1a2 polymorphism on the ergogenic effects of caffeine. J Int Soc Sports Nutr 2012, 9:7.
54. Del Coso J, Salinero JJ, Gonzalez-Millan C, et al.: Dose response effects of a caffeine-containing energy drink on muscle performance: A repeated measures design. J Int Soc Sports Nutr 2012, 9:21.
55. Ratamess NA, Bush JA, Kang J, et al.: The effects of supplementation with p-synephrine alone and in combination with caffeine on resistance exercise performance. J Int Soc Sports Nutr 2015, 12:35.
56. Richardson DL and Clarke ND: Effect of coffee and caffeine ingestion on resistance exercise performance. J Strength Cond Res 2016.
57. Trexler ET, Smith-Ryan AE, Roelofs EJ, et al.: Effects of coffee and caffeine anhydrous on strength and sprint performance. Eur J Sport Sci 2016, 16:702-10.
58. Kerksick C, Harvey T, Stout J, et al.: International society of sports nutrition position stand: Nutrient timing. J Int Soc Sports Nutr 2008, 5:17.
59. Flakoll PJ, Judy T, Flinn K, et al.: Postexercise protein supplementation improves health and muscle soreness during basic military training in marine recruits. J Appl Physiol (1985) 2004, 96:951-6.
60. Areta JL, Burke LM, Ross ML, et al.: Timing and distribution of protein ingestion during prolonged recovery from resistance exercise alters myofibrillar protein synthesis. J Physiol 2013, 591:2319-31.
61. Kanda A, Nakayama K, Sanbongi C, et al.: Effects of whey, caseinate, or milk protein ingestion on muscle protein synthesis after exercise. Nutrients 2016, 8.
62. Levine JA, Vander Weg MW, Hill JO, et al.: Non-exercise activity thermogenesis: The crouching tiger hidden dragon of societal weight gain. Arterioscler

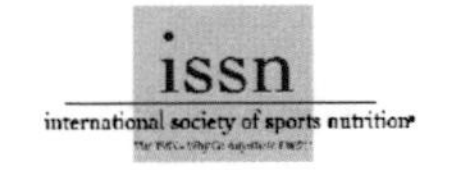

Thromb Vasc Biol 2006, 26:729-36.
63. Wycherley TP, Buckley JD, Noakes M, et al.: Long-term effects of a very low-carbohydrate weight loss diet on exercise capacity and tolerance in overweight and obese adults. J Am Coll Nutr 2014, 33:267-73.
64. Mansour MS, Ni YM, Roberts AL, et al.: Ginger consumption enhances the thermic effect of food and promotes feelings of satiety without affecting metabolic and hormonal parameters in overweight men: A pilot study. Metabolism 2012, 61:1347-52.
65. Sutton EF, Bray GA, Burton JH, et al.: No evidence for metabolic adaptation in thermic effect of food by dietary protein. Obesity (Silver Spring) 2016, 24:1639-42.
66. Farshchi HR, Taylor MA, and Macdonald IA: Decreased thermic effect of food after an irregular compared with a regular meal pattern in healthy lean women. Int J Obes Relat Metab Disord 2004, 28:653-60.
67. Hall KD, Chen KY, Guo J, et al.: Energy expenditure and body composition changes after an isocaloric ketogenic diet in overweight and obese men. Am J Clin Nutr 2016, 104:324-33.
68. Baum JI, Gray M, and Binns A: Breakfasts higher in protein increase postprandial energy expenditure, increase fat oxidation, and reduce hunger in overweight children from 8 to 12 years of age. J Nutr 2015, 145:2229-35.
69. Longland TM, Oikawa SY, Mitchell CJ, et al.: Higher compared with lower dietary protein during an energy deficit combined with intense exercise promotes greater lean mass gain and fat mass loss: A randomized trial. Am J Clin Nutr 2016, 103:738-46.
70. Thomson RL, Brinkworth GD, Noakes M, et al.: Muscle strength gains during resistance exercise training are attenuated with soy compared with dairy or usual protein intake in older adults: A randomized controlled trial. Clin Nutr 2016, 35:27-33.
71. Loftfield E, Freedman ND, Graubard BI, et al.: Association of coffee consumption with overall and

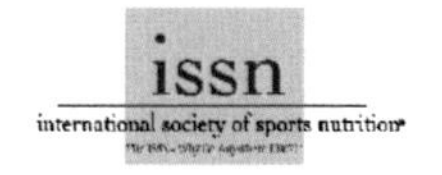

cause-specific mortality in a large us prospective cohort study. Am J Epidemiol 2015, 182:1010-22.

72. Liebeskind DS, Sanossian N, Fu KA, et al.: The coffee paradox in stroke: Increased consumption linked with fewer strokes. Nutr Neurosci 2015.
73. Clifford T, Bell O, West DJ, et al.: The effects of beetroot juice supplementation on indices of muscle damage following eccentric exercise. Eur J Appl Physiol 2016, 116:353-62.
74. Muggeridge DJ, Howe CC, Spendiff O, et al.: A single dose of beetroot juice enhances cycling performance in simulated altitude. Med Sci Sports Exerc 2014, 46:143-50.
75. Josse AR, Tang JE, Tarnopolsky MA, et al.: Body composition and strength changes in women with milk and resistance exercise. Med Sci Sports Exerc 2010, 42:1122-30.
76. Patel RK, Brouner J, and Spendiff O: Dark chocolate supplementation reduces the oxygen cost of moderate intensity cycling. J Int Soc Sports Nutr 2015, 12:47.
77. Li B, Zhang G, Tan M, et al.: Consumption of whole grains in relation to mortality from all causes, cardiovascular disease, and diabetes: Dose-response meta-analysis of prospective cohort studies. Medicine (Baltimore) 2016, 95:e4229.
78. Hill AM, Buckley JD, Murphy KJ, et al.: Combining fish-oil supplements with regular aerobic exercise improves body composition and cardiovascular disease risk factors. Am J Clin Nutr 2007, 85:1267-74.
79. Jimenez-Pavon D, Cervantes-Borunda MS, Diaz LE, et al.: Effects of a moderate intake of beer on markers of hydration after exercise in the heat: A crossover study. J Int Soc Sports Nutr 2015, 12:26.
80. Djousse L, Hopkins PN, North KE, et al.: Chocolate consumption is inversely associated with prevalent coronary heart disease: The national heart, lung, and blood institute family heart study. Clin Nutr 2011, 30:182-7.
81. Saito E, Inoue M, Sawada N, et al.: Association of

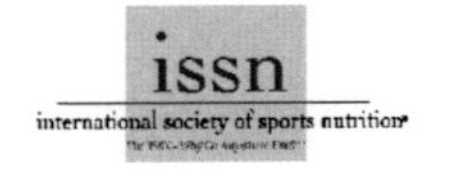

green tea consumption with mortality due to all causes and major causes of death in a japanese population: The japan public health center-based prospective study (jphc study). Ann Epidemiol 2015, 25:512-518 e3.

82. Peeling P, Cox GR, Bullock N, et al.: Beetroot juice improves on-water 500 m time-trial performance, and laboratory-based paddling economy in national and international-level kayak athletes. Int J Sport Nutr Exerc Metab 2015, 25:278-84.
83. Arnold JT, Oliver SJ, Lewis-Jones TM, et al.: Beetroot juice does not enhance altitude running performance in well-trained athletes. Appl Physiol Nutr Metab 2015, 40:590-5.
84. Grant MC and Baker JS: An overview of the effect of probiotics and exercise on mood and associated health conditions. Crit Rev Food Sci Nutr 2016:0.
85. Shing CM, Peake JM, Lim CL, et al.: Effects of probiotics supplementation on gastrointestinal permeability, inflammation and exercise performance in the heat. Eur J Appl Physiol 2014, 114:93-103.
86. Trepanowski JF, Farney TM, McCarthy CG, et al.: The effects of chronic betaine supplementation on exercise performance, skeletal muscle oxygen saturation and associated biochemical parameters in resistance trained men. J Strength Cond Res 2011, 25:3461-71.
87. van Rosendal SP, Osborne MA, Fassett RG, et al.: Guidelines for glycerol use in hyperhydration and rehydration associated with exercise. Sports Med 2010, 40:113-29.
88. Hoffman JR, Stout JR, Williams DR, et al.: Efficacy of phosphatidic acid ingestion on lean body mass, muscle thickness and strength gains in resistance-trained men. J Int Soc Sports Nutr 2012, 9:47.
89. Legault Z, Bagnall N, and Kimmerly DS: The influence of oral l-glutamine supplementation on muscle strength recovery and soreness following unilateral knee extension eccentric exercise. Int J Sport Nutr

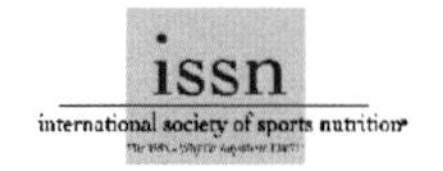

Exerc Metab 2015, 25:417-26.
90. Bellar D, LeBlanc NR, and Campbell B: The effect of 6 days of alpha glycerylphosphorylcholine on isometric strength. J Int Soc Sports Nutr 2015, 12:42.
91. Kingsley MI, Miller M, Kilduff LP, et al.: Effects of phosphatidylserine on exercise capacity during cycling in active males. Med Sci Sports Exerc 2006, 38:64-71.
92. McCormack WP, Hoffman JR, Pruna GJ, et al.: Effects of l-alanyl-l-glutamine ingestion on one-hour run performance. J Am Coll Nutr 2015, 34:488-96.
93. De Souza EO, Lowery RP, Wilson JM, et al.: Effects of arachidonic acid supplementation on acute anabolic signaling and chronic functional performance and body composition adaptations. PLoS One 2016, 11:e0155153.
94. Pirbaglou M, Katz J, de Souza RJ, et al.: Probiotic supplementation can positively affect anxiety and depressive symptoms: A systematic review of randomized controlled trials. Nutr Res 2016, 36:889-98.
95. Trexler ET, Smith-Ryan AE, Stout JR, et al.: International society of sports nutrition position stand: Beta-alanine. J Int Soc Sports Nutr 2015, 12:30.
96. Smith AE, Walter AA, Graef JL, et al.: Effects of beta-alanine supplementation and high-intensity interval training on endurance performance and body composition in men; a double-blind trial. J Int Soc Sports Nutr 2009, 6:5.
97. Hobson RM, Harris RC, Martin D, et al.: Effect of beta-alanine, with and without sodium bicarbonate, on 2000-m rowing performance. Int J Sport Nutr Exerc Metab 2013, 23:480-7.
98. Bellinger PM and Minahan CL: The effect of beta-alanine supplementation on cycling time trials of different length. Eur J Sport Sci 2016, 16:829-36.
99. Hoffman JR, Landau G, Stout JR, et al.: Beta-alanine supplementation improves tactical performance but not cognitive function in combat soldiers. J Int Soc Sports Nutr 2014, 11:15.

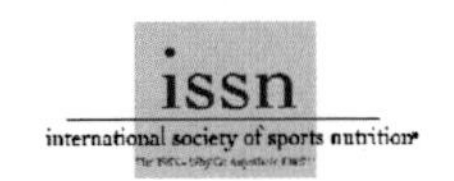

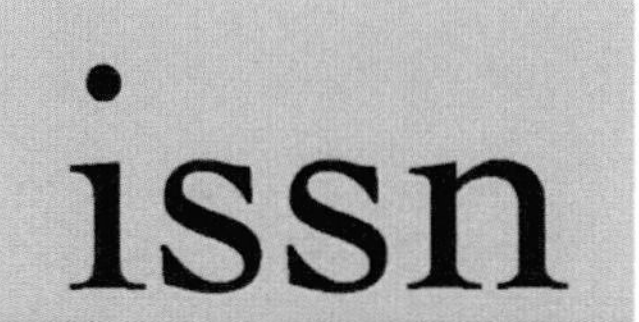

international society of sports nutrition®

The ISSN – Why Go Anywhere Else?!™

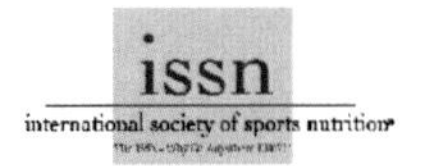

Made in the USA
Middletown, DE
08 December 2019

80273619R00042